BLACK SEED OIL FOR CANCER TREATMENT

Unlocking Nature's Potential: A Comprehensive Guide to Black Seed Oil's Role in Cancer Support and Beyond

DR. PAUL VANJAY

Black Seed Oil For Cancer Treatment

INTRODUCTION

Cancer is a devastating disease that affects millions of people worldwide. Despite advancements in conventional cancer treatments, many patients still suffer from the harsh side effects of chemotherapy, radiation therapy, and other conventional therapies. As a result, there has been a growing interest in alternative and complementary therapies that can help improve cancer patients' quality of life and possibly even enhance their treatment outcomes.

Black seed oil is a natural substance that has been used for centuries to treat a variety of health conditions, including cancer. It is extracted from the seeds of the Nigella Sativa plant, which is native to the Middle East and North Africa. Black seed oil has gained popularity in recent years due to its potential health benefits, and its use as a complementary treatment for cancer is a topic of ongoing research.

This book aims to provide a comprehensive overview of black seed oil and its potential as a complementary treatment for cancer. We will explore the science behind black seed oil and its active compounds, as well as its potential interactions with conventional cancer treatments. We will also examine the evidence for the effectiveness of black seed oil in cancer treatment and its potential benefits and side effects. Additionally, we will share personal stories of cancer patients who have used black seed oil as a complementary treatment, and discuss the role of black seed oil in integrative oncology.

By the end of this book, you will have a better understanding of black seed oil's potential as a complementary treatment for cancer and its place in integrative cancer care. We hope that this book will inspire further research and education on alternative and complementary cancer treatments and help cancer patients make informed decisions about their health and well-being.

UNDERSTANDING CANCER: AN OVERVIEW

Cancer is a complex and multifaceted group of diseases characterized by the uncontrolled growth and spread of abnormal cells. This condition, which can affect virtually any tissue or organ in the body, arises from genetic mutations that disrupt the normal regulatory mechanisms of the cell cycle. In a healthy organism, cells undergo a tightly regulated process of growth, division, and programmed death. However, when the intricate balance of this cycle is disrupted, uncontrolled cell growth can lead to the formation of tumors.

Key Concepts in Cancer Biology:

1. **Genetic Mutations:**

   - **Initiation of Cancer:** Genetic mutations, whether inherited or acquired, play a pivotal role in the initiation of cancer. These mutations can be caused by various factors, including exposure to carcinogens, genetic predisposition, or random errors during cell division.

2. **Cell Cycle Aberrations:**

   - **Dysregulation:** Cancer cells often exhibit dysregulation in the cell cycle, allowing them to continuously divide and evade normal cell death processes. This uncontrolled growth forms the basis of tumor development.

3. **Tumor Types:**

   - **Benign vs. Malignant:** Tumors are classified as benign or malignant based on their behavior. Benign tumors are usually non-invasive and do not spread, while malignant tumors have the potential to invade surrounding tissues and metastasize to distant organs.

4. **Metastasis:**

- **Spreading Beyond:** Cancer becomes particularly challenging when cells acquire the ability to metastasize—traveling through the bloodstream or lymphatic system to form secondary tumors in distant parts of the body. Metastasis often signifies advanced disease stages and complicates treatment strategies.

Types of Cancer

1. **Breast Cancer:**

    - Originates in the cells of the breast tissue, most commonly in the milk ducts or lobules. It affects both men and women.

2. **Lung Cancer:**

    - Primarily associated with the lungs, lung cancer is often linked to smoking but can also occur in non-smokers.

3. **Colorectal Cancer:**

    - Affects the colon or rectum and usually develops from precancerous polyps. It includes colon cancer and rectal cancer.

4. **Prostate Cancer:**

- Occurs in the prostate, a small walnut-shaped gland in men that produces seminal fluid.

5. **Ovarian Cancer:**

   - Originates in the ovaries, which are part of the female reproductive system.

6. **Leukemia:**

   - A type of blood cancer that affects the bone marrow and blood. It is characterized by the rapid production of abnormal white blood cells.

7. **Lymphoma:**

   - A cancer that begins in the lymphatic system, which is part of the immune system. There are two main types:

Black Seed Oil For Cancer Treatment

Hodgkin lymphoma and non-Hodgkin lymphoma.

8. **Melanoma:**

- Arises in the pigment-producing cells (melanocytes) of the skin. It is a type of skin cancer that can spread to other parts of the body.

9. **Pancreatic Cancer:**

- Develops in the pancreas, an organ that produces digestive enzymes and hormones like insulin.

10. **Bladder Cancer:**

- Affects the bladder, which is part of the urinary system. It often starts in the cells lining the bladder.

11. **Kidney Cancer:**

  - Originates in the kidneys, vital organs that filter waste products from the blood to form urine.

12. **Liver Cancer:**

  - Primarily associated with hepatocellular carcinoma and often develops in individuals with chronic liver disease.

13. **Brain Tumors:**

  - Tumors that can be benign or malignant and develop in the brain or spinal cord.

14. **Thyroid Cancer:**

  - Affects the thyroid gland, a butterfly-shaped organ in the neck that produces hormones.

15. **Esophageal Cancer:**

- Occurs in the esophagus, the tube that carries food from the mouth to the stomach.

16. **Stomach (Gastric) Cancer:**

- Develops in the lining of the stomach and is often associated with certain risk factors such as infection with Helicobacter pylori.

17. **Cervical Cancer:**

- Affects the cervix, the lower part of the uterus, and is often associated with human papillomavirus (HPV) infection.

Understanding the specific type of cancer is crucial for determining the most effective treatment approaches and developing personalized care plans for individuals diagnosed with the disease.

Causes of cancer

Cancer is a complex disease, and its development is often influenced by a combination of genetic, environmental, and lifestyle factors. While the exact causes of cancer can vary depending on the type of cancer, some common factors contribute to the initiation and progression of the disease. Here are key factors associated with the development of cancer:

1. **Genetic Factors:**

    - **Inherited Mutations:** Some individuals inherit genetic mutations that predispose them to certain types of cancer. These mutations can be passed down from parents to their children and increase the risk of developing cancer.

2. **Environmental Exposures:**

   - **Carcinogens:** Exposure to certain substances known as carcinogens increases the risk of cancer. Examples include tobacco smoke, asbestos, certain chemicals, and pollutants.

3. **Lifestyle Choices:**

   - **Tobacco Use:** Smoking and the use of tobacco products are leading causes of various cancers, particularly lung, throat, and mouth cancers.

   - **Diet:** Poor dietary choices, such as a high intake of processed foods, red meat, and low consumption of fruits and vegetables, can contribute to cancer risk.

- **Alcohol Consumption:** Excessive alcohol consumption has been linked to an increased risk of several cancers, including liver, breast, and colorectal cancer.

- **Physical Inactivity:** Lack of regular physical activity is associated with an elevated risk of certain cancers.

4. **Infections:**

- **Viral Infections:** Infections with certain viruses, bacteria, and parasites can increase the risk of specific cancers. Examples include human papillomavirus (HPV) and cervical cancer, hepatitis B and C viruses and liver cancer, and Helicobacter pylori and stomach cancer.

5. **Radiation Exposure:**

- **Ionizing Radiation:** Prolonged exposure to ionizing radiation, such as X-rays and certain occupational exposures, can increase the risk of cancer.

6. **Hormonal Factors:**

- **Hormone Replacement Therapy (HRT):** Long-term use of hormone replacement therapy in postmenopausal women has been associated with an increased risk of certain cancers.

- **Reproductive and Menstrual Factors:** Early onset of menstruation, late onset of menopause, and nulliparity (not having children) can influence the risk of breast and ovarian cancers.

7. **Chronic Inflammation:**

- **Inflammatory Conditions:** Chronic inflammatory conditions, such as inflammatory bowel disease (e.g., Crohn's disease, ulcerative colitis), are associated with an increased risk of developing certain cancers.

8. **Age and Genetics:**

- **Age:** The risk of cancer generally increases with age, as genetic mutations accumulate over time.

- **Gender and Ethnicity:** Some types of cancer are more common in specific genders or ethnic groups.

It's important to note that the development of cancer is often multifactorial, involving the interplay of various risk factors. Additionally, not everyone exposed to these risk factors will develop cancer, and individuals without apparent risk factors may still be diagnosed with the disease. Regular screenings, a healthy lifestyle, and early detection can significantly contribute to cancer prevention and improved outcomes.

Risk factors

Risk factors are conditions or behaviors that increase the likelihood of developing a particular disease, in this case, cancer. Understanding these risk factors is crucial for prevention, early detection, and developing strategies to reduce the overall risk of cancer. Here are common risk factors associated with cancer:

1. **Age:**

   - The risk of cancer generally increases with age. Many cancers are diagnosed in individuals over the age of 65.

2. **Genetic Factors:**

   - **Inherited Mutations:** Some individuals carry genetic mutations inherited from their parents, increasing their susceptibility to certain types of cancer.

   - **Family History:** A family history of certain cancers may indicate a genetic predisposition to the disease.

3. **Environmental Exposures:**

   - **Carcinogens:** Exposure to substances known as carcinogens, such as tobacco smoke, asbestos, and certain chemicals, can elevate cancer risk.

4. **Lifestyle Choices:**

   - **Tobacco Use:** Smoking and the use of tobacco products are major risk factors for various cancers, including lung, throat, and mouth cancers.

   - **Dietary Habits:** A diet high in processed foods, red meat, and low in fruits and vegetables may contribute to cancer risk.

   - **Alcohol Consumption:** Excessive alcohol consumption increases the risk of several cancers, including liver, breast, and colorectal cancer.

- **Physical Inactivity:** Lack of regular exercise is associated with an increased risk of certain cancers.

5. **Infections:**

- **Viral Infections:** Infections with certain viruses, such as human papillomavirus (HPV), hepatitis B and C, and human immunodeficiency virus (HIV), are linked to specific cancers.

6. **Hormonal Factors:**

- **Hormone Replacement Therapy (HRT):** Long-term use of hormone replacement therapy in postmenopausal women may increase the risk of certain cancers.

- **Reproductive Factors:** Early menstruation, late menopause, and nulliparity (not having children) can influence the risk of breast and ovarian cancers.

7. **Radiation Exposure:**

- **Ionizing Radiation:** Prolonged exposure to ionizing radiation, such as medical X-rays or certain occupational exposures, can increase cancer risk.

8. **Chronic Inflammation:**

- **Inflammatory Conditions:** Chronic inflammatory conditions, such as inflammatory bowel disease (e.g.,

Crohn's disease, ulcerative colitis), are associated with an increased risk of certain cancers.

9. **Obesity:**

- Being overweight or obese is a risk factor for several cancers, including breast, colorectal, and endometrial cancers.

10. **Sun Exposure:**

- Prolonged exposure to ultraviolet (UV) radiation from the sun or tanning beds increases the risk of skin cancer, including melanoma.

11. **Occupational Exposures:**

- Certain occupational exposures to chemicals, toxins, and pollutants may contribute to an increased risk of cancer.

12. **Gender and Ethnicity:**

- Some types of cancer are more prevalent in specific genders or ethnic groups.

It's important to note that having one or more risk factors doesn't guarantee the development of cancer, and individuals without apparent risk factors can still be diagnosed with the disease. Regular screenings, adopting a healthy lifestyle, and awareness of one's family and personal medical history are essential in managing and mitigating cancer risk.

Complications

Cancer can lead to various complications, both as a result of the disease itself and the treatments employed to manage it. The complications can vary widely depending on the type and stage of cancer, as well as the individual's overall health. Here are some common complications associated with cancer:

1. **Spread (Metastasis):**

   - One of the primary complications of cancer is the spread of cancer cells to other parts of the body, a process known as metastasis. This can make treatment more challenging and affect multiple organ systems.

2. **Side Effects of Treatment:**

- **Chemotherapy Side Effects:** Chemotherapy drugs, while effective in killing cancer cells, can also harm healthy cells, leading to side effects such as nausea, fatigue, hair loss, and increased susceptibility to infections.

- **Radiation Side Effects:** Radiation therapy may cause side effects depending on the area being treated, including skin changes, fatigue, and damage to surrounding tissues.

- **Immunotherapy Side Effects:** Immunotherapy, while harnessing the immune system to fight cancer, can lead to immune-related side effects, such as inflammation of organs or autoimmune reactions.

3. **Compromised Immune System:**

- Cancer and certain cancer treatments can weaken the immune system, making individuals more susceptible to infections and other illnesses.

4. **Pain:**

- Cancer itself or its treatment may cause pain. Pain can be localized to the tumor site or may be a result of nerve damage or inflammation.

5. **Blood-related Complications:**

- **Anemia:** Cancer and cancer treatments can lead to a decrease in red blood cells, causing fatigue and weakness.

- **Thrombocytopenia:** A reduction in platelets, essential for blood clotting, can result in an increased risk of bleeding and bruising.

6. **Emotional and Psychological Effects:**

- The emotional toll of cancer can be significant, leading to anxiety, depression, and stress. Coping with the uncertainty of the disease and the impact on daily life can contribute to mental health challenges.

7. **Nutritional Challenges:**

Black Seed Oil For Cancer Treatment

- Cancer can affect appetite, and some treatments may cause nausea or difficulty eating, leading to weight loss and malnutrition.

8. **Hormonal Changes:**

- Certain cancers, such as breast or prostate cancer, can affect hormone levels, leading to a range of symptoms and complications.

9. **Cognitive Changes:**

- Some cancer patients may experience cognitive changes, often referred to as "chemo brain," characterized by memory lapses, difficulty concentrating, and mental fogginess.

10. **Secondary Cancers:**

- Certain cancer treatments, especially radiation therapy and some chemotherapy drugs, may increase the risk of developing secondary cancers later in life.

11. Financial and Social Impact:

- The financial burden of cancer treatment, coupled with potential disruptions to work and social life, can contribute to stress and strain on relationships.

12. Treatment-related Long-term Effects:

- Some cancer survivors may experience long-term effects of treatment, known as late effects, which can impact organ function or overall health.

It's important for individuals with cancer to work closely with their healthcare team to manage and mitigate these complications. Support from healthcare professionals, family, and support groups can play a crucial role in addressing the various challenges associated with cancer and its treatments.

Diagnosis

The diagnosis of cancer involves a thorough process that combines various medical techniques and tests to identify the presence of abnormal cells or tumors. Timely and accurate diagnosis is crucial for determining the type, stage, and characteristics of the cancer, which then guides the development of an appropriate treatment plan. Here are key components of the cancer diagnosis process:

1. Medical History and Physical Examination:

- **Patient Interview:** Gathering information about the patient's personal and family medical history, lifestyle factors, and any symptoms they may be experiencing.

- **Physical Examination:** A comprehensive physical examination to detect any abnormalities, such as lumps or changes in organ size.

2. Diagnostic Imaging:

- **X-rays, CT Scans, and MRI:** Imaging techniques provide detailed pictures of the internal structures, helping to identify tumors, their size, and their location.

- **Ultrasound:** Uses sound waves to create images, often employed to visualize organs and tissues.

- **PET Scans:** Positron Emission Tomography scans can reveal metabolic activity in tissues, aiding in cancer detection.

3. Biopsy:

- **Tissue Sampling:** A biopsy involves the removal of a small sample of tissue for examination under a microscope. This definitive test confirms the presence of cancer, determines its type, and provides information about its characteristics.

4. Blood Tests:

- **Tumor Markers:** Blood tests can detect certain substances produced by cancer cells, known as tumor markers. Elevated levels may indicate the presence of cancer, but they are not conclusive and often require further investigation.

5. Endoscopy:

- **Direct Visualization:** Endoscopic procedures allow doctors to directly visualize the inside of organs using a flexible tube with a light and camera. Common examples include colonoscopy, bronchoscopy, and upper endoscopy.

6. Bone Marrow Aspiration and Biopsy:

- **Blood Cell Production:** In cases of blood cancers or metastatic cancers, samples of bone marrow may be taken to assess the health of blood cell production.

7. Genetic Testing:

- **Identifying Mutations:** Genetic tests can identify specific mutations or alterations in genes that may increase the risk of developing certain types of cancer or influence treatment decisions.

8. Lymph Node Biopsy:

- **Spread Assessment:** If cancer has spread, a biopsy of nearby lymph nodes may be performed to determine the extent of metastasis.

9. Histopathology and Cytology:

- **Microscopic Examination:** Pathologists examine tissue and cell samples under a microscope to determine the type and characteristics of cancer cells.

10. Molecular Profiling:

- **Tumor Molecular Characteristics:** Molecular profiling analyzes the genetic makeup of tumors to identify specific mutations. This information can guide targeted therapies.

11. Staging:

- **Determining Extent:** Staging involves assessing the size of the tumor, its spread to nearby tissues or lymph nodes, and, if applicable, its metastasis to other parts of the body. Staging helps determine the prognosis and appropriate treatment.

12. Multidisciplinary Consultation:

- **Collaborative Decision-Making:** Oncologists, surgeons, radiologists, pathologists, and other specialists collaborate to review all diagnostic information and formulate a comprehensive treatment plan.

A precise and comprehensive diagnosis is foundational for developing an effective and tailored treatment approach. Advances in diagnostic technologies and personalized medicine continue to enhance the accuracy and precision of cancer diagnoses.

Conventional Cancer Treatments:

1. **Surgery:**

    - **Primary Intervention:** Surgery involves the physical removal of tumors and is often the primary treatment for localized cancers. Its efficacy depends on factors such as tumor size, location, and accessibility.

2. **Chemotherapy:**

    - **Cellular Targeting:** Chemotherapy employs drugs that target rapidly dividing cells, including cancer cells. However, it can affect normal cells as well, leading to side effects such as hair loss, nausea, and fatigue.

3. **Radiation Therapy:**

- **Precision in Targeting:** Radiation therapy utilizes high doses of radiation to damage or destroy cancer cells. Precise targeting is crucial to spare surrounding healthy tissues from harm.

4. **Immunotherapy:**

- **Harnessing the Immune System:** Immunotherapy works by enhancing the body's immune response against cancer cells. This novel approach has shown promise in treating certain types of cancer.

The Need for Alternative Approaches:

1. **Side Effects:**

- **Impact on Quality of Life:** Conventional treatments often come with significant side effects that can affect a patient's well-being and quality of life. This has spurred interest in alternative and complementary approaches that may mitigate these effects.

2. **Resistant Strains:**

   - **Adaptation and Resistance:** Some cancers develop resistance to standard treatments over time, necessitating the exploration of innovative therapeutic strategies.

3. **Holistic Care:**

   - **Addressing the Whole Patient:** Recognizing cancer as not only a physical ailment but also an emotional and psychological challenge emphasizes the importance of holistic patient-centered care.

4. **Integrative Medicine:**

- **Combining Approaches:** Integrative medicine seeks to combine conventional and alternative therapies to provide a comprehensive and personalized approach to cancer treatment.

In the ongoing pursuit of understanding and treating cancer, a multi-faceted approach that integrates advances in conventional medicine with insights from alternative and complementary practices holds promise for improving outcomes and enhancing the overall well-being of individuals facing this formidable challenge.

Integrative Oncology and its Principles

Integrative oncology is a field that combines conventional cancer treatments with complementary therapies, such as acupuncture, massage, and nutrition counseling. The goal of integrative oncology is to provide a comprehensive approach to cancer care that addresses not only the physical aspects of the disease, but also the emotional, social, and spiritual needs of patients.

The principles of integrative oncology include:

- Patient-centered care: focusing on the needs and preferences of individual patients

- Collaboration: involving a team of healthcare professionals who work together to provide comprehensive care

- Evidence-based practice: using the best available research to guide treatment decisions

- Safety: prioritizing the safety of patients and avoiding harm

- Personalization: tailoring treatment plans to the unique needs and circumstances of each patient

The Role of Black Seed Oil in Integrative Cancer Care

Black seed oil may have a role to play in integrative cancer care. Research has suggested that black seed oil may have anti-cancer properties, and may also have benefits such as reducing inflammation and boosting the immune system.

Black seed oil may be used in conjunction with conventional cancer treatments, such as chemotherapy and radiation therapy, as a way to mitigate side effects and improve quality of life. It may also be used as a standalone therapy for patients who are seeking complementary or alternative treatments.

BLACK SEED OIL: A COMPREHENSIVE OVERVIEW

Black seed oil is a natural oil extracted from the seeds of the Nigella Sativa plant. It is also known as black cumin oil, kalonji oil, or black caraway oil. Black seed oil has been used for centuries in traditional medicine to treat a variety of ailments, including digestive disorders, respiratory conditions, and skin problems.

Historical Background of Black Seed Oil

Black seed oil, derived from the seeds of Nigella sativa, holds a rich historical background deeply embedded in various cultures and civilizations. Known by different names such as black cumin, black caraway, and kalonji, black seed oil has been prized for its culinary, medicinal, and symbolic significance throughout history.

Ancient Egypt:

- **Ancient Remedies:** Black seed oil has roots dating back to ancient Egypt, where it was discovered in the tomb of King Tutankhamun. Egyptians regarded it so highly that they believed it could accompany the deceased in the afterlife.

- **Culinary and Medicinal Uses:** In addition to its symbolic importance, black seed was used in culinary practices and as a traditional remedy for various ailments.

Middle East and Islamic Civilization:

- **Prophetic Mention:** Black seed oil gained prominence in Islamic traditions due to its mention in various hadiths (sayings of Prophet

Muhammad). It is often referred to as "Habbat al-Barakah" (the blessed seed).

- **Traditional Medicine:** Islamic scholars and physicians, including Avicenna (Ibn Sina), highlighted the medicinal properties of black seed oil in their writings. It became a staple in traditional Middle Eastern medicine.

Ancient Greece and Rome:

- **Hippocrates and Dioscorides:** Even in ancient Greece, renowned figures like Hippocrates, the "father of medicine," and Dioscorides, a physician and pharmacologist, recognized the therapeutic potential of black seed. They used it for digestive and respiratory issues.

Indian Ayurveda and Traditional Chinese Medicine:

- **Ayurvedic Practices:** In India, black seed was embraced in Ayurvedic practices, believed to balance the three doshas (Vata, Pitta, Kapha) and support overall well-being.

- **TCM Incorporation:** Traditional Chinese Medicine (TCM) also incorporated black seed for its purported medicinal properties, emphasizing its role in balancing bodily energies.

Medieval and Renaissance Europe:

- **Spices and Trade:** During the medieval period, black seed became a sought-after spice and medicinal herb. Its popularity in trade routes contributed to its spread across Europe.

- **Monastic Gardens:** Monastic gardens in Europe often cultivated black seed for both culinary and medicinal purposes.

Modern Rediscovery:

- **Scientific Interest:** In the 20th century, scientific interest in black seed oil began to rise. Researchers started exploring its chemical composition and potential health benefits.

- **Contemporary Uses:** Today, black seed oil is available worldwide, often used as a dietary supplement, in skincare products, and explored for its potential therapeutic applications in modern medicine.

BLACK SEED OIL FOR CANCER TREATMENT

While research on the use of black seed oil in cancer treatment is still in its early stages, there is potential for future research and development in this field. Further studies could explore the mechanisms of action of black seed oil, optimal dosages and administration methods, and potential interactions with other medications.

In addition, more research could be conducted on the use of black seed oil in integrative oncology. For example, studies could investigate the use of black seed oil in combination with other complementary therapies, or in specific patient populations such as those with advanced cancer or those undergoing palliative care.

Black seed oil may have a role to play in integrative oncology as a complementary therapy for cancer patients. As research in this field continues to evolve, there may be opportunities for black seed oil to be integrated into cancer treatment plans in new and innovative ways.

While black seed oil has been traditionally used for various health purposes and is being researched for its potential benefits, it's crucial to approach claims about its efficacy in cancer treatment with caution.

Here's an overview:

Limited Scientific Evidence:

1. **Lab Studies:** Some laboratory studies suggest that certain compounds in black seed oil, such as thymoquinone, may have anti-cancer

properties by affecting cancer cell proliferation and apoptosis.

2. **Animal Studies:** Animal studies have shown some promising results, but the transition from animal studies to human applications requires careful consideration.

Clinical Studies and Human Trials:

1. **Insufficient Data:** There is a lack of well-designed clinical trials and large-scale human studies to establish the effectiveness of black seed oil in preventing or treating cancer in humans.

2. **Heterogeneity of Studies:** Existing studies often differ in methodologies, doses, and formulations, making it challenging to draw definitive conclusions.

Black Seed Oil For Cancer Treatment

Cautions and Considerations:

1. **Consultation with Healthcare Professionals:** Individuals considering alternative or complementary treatments, including black seed oil, should consult with their healthcare professionals. It's important to discuss any plans to incorporate such substances into a cancer treatment regimen.

2. **Safety Concerns:** While black seed oil is generally considered safe for culinary use and as a supplement in moderate amounts, high doses may lead to potential side effects. It may also interact with certain medications.

Holistic Approach and Integrative Medicine:

1. **Supplemental Role:** If considered, black seed oil might be explored as part of a holistic

approach to cancer care, complementing conventional treatments rather than replacing them.

2. **Patient-Centered Care:** Integrative medicine focuses on patient-centered care, emphasizing the importance of overall well-being and quality of life during cancer treatment.

While there's ongoing interest in the potential health benefits of black seed oil, especially in preclinical studies, more rigorous research is needed to establish its role in cancer treatment. Cancer patients should rely on evidence-based conventional treatments, and any complementary approaches should be discussed thoroughly with healthcare professionals.

For the latest and more specific information, it is advisable to consult recent medical literature or speak directly with healthcare providers who can provide guidance based on the most current research and understanding.

Other Health Benefits of Black Seed Oil

1. Anti-Inflammatory Properties:

- **Compounds such as thymoquinone in black seed oil are believed to have anti-inflammatory effects,** which may be beneficial for conditions involving inflammation.

2. Antioxidant Effects:

- **Black seed oil contains antioxidants that help neutralize free radicals,** potentially reducing oxidative stress in the body.

Black Seed Oil For Cancer Treatment

3. Immune System Support:

- **Studies suggest that black seed oil may have immunomodulatory effects,** potentially enhancing the body's natural defenses.

4. Respiratory Health:

- **Traditional uses include remedies for respiratory conditions,** and some studies suggest potential benefits in conditions like asthma and allergies.

5. Cardiovascular Health:

- **Some research indicates that black seed oil may positively impact cholesterol levels and blood pressure,** contributing to cardiovascular health.

- **Anti-atherogenic properties may reduce the risk of atherosclerosis.**

6. Diabetes Management:

- **Preliminary studies suggest that black seed oil may aid in managing blood sugar levels,** offering potential benefits for individuals with diabetes.

- **Improved insulin sensitivity has been observed in some studies.**

7. Skin Conditions:

- **Topical application of black seed oil is believed to benefit various skin conditions,** including acne, eczema, and psoriasis, due to its anti-inflammatory and antimicrobial properties.

8. Gastrointestinal Health:

- **Black seed oil has been traditionally used to aid digestion,** and some studies suggest potential benefits in gastrointestinal conditions.

9. Pain Management:

- **Anti-inflammatory properties may contribute to the alleviation of certain types of pain,** although more research is needed in this area.

10. Weight Management:

- **Some studies suggest that black seed oil may have a role in weight management,** potentially reducing body weight and improving metabolic parameters.

11. Cognitive Function:

- **Preliminary research has explored the potential neuroprotective effects of black seed oil,** indicating possible benefits for cognitive function.

12. Antimicrobial Properties:

- **Black seed oil has demonstrated antimicrobial effects,** suggesting potential benefits against various pathogens.

13. Menstrual Health:

- **Traditional use includes the use of black seed oil for menstrual health,** although scientific evidence in this area is limited.

14. Hair and Scalp Health:

- **Topical application of black seed oil is believed to strengthen hair and promote a healthy scalp,** although individual responses may vary.

Cautions:

- **Dosage and Individual Responses:** The effectiveness of black seed oil may vary among individuals, and proper dosage is essential.

- **Interactions:** Individuals taking medications or with existing health conditions should consult with healthcare professionals, as black seed oil may interact with certain medications.

Dosage and preparation

The dosage and preparation of black seed oil can vary depending on the intended use and individual factors.

It's important to note that while black seed oil is

generally considered safe for many people, there is no established standard dosage, and individual responses can vary. Here are general guidelines for dosage and preparation:

1. Dosage:

- **Oral Consumption:** For general health and well-being, a common recommendation is to take about one to two teaspoons (approximately 5-10 mL) of black seed oil per day.

- **Specific Health Conditions:** If using black seed oil for a specific health condition or concern, the dosage may vary. It's advisable to consult with a healthcare professional to determine an appropriate and personalized dosage.

**2. Preparation:

- **Pure Oil:** High-quality, pure black seed oil is typically recommended. Look for oil extracted from organic, non-GMO Nigella sativa seeds.

- **Cold-Pressed:** Cold-pressed oils are preferred, as this method helps preserve the beneficial compounds in the oil.

- **Storage:** Store black seed oil in a cool, dark place, away from direct sunlight, to prevent degradation of its quality.

- **Mixing with Other Substances:** Some people mix black seed oil with honey, yogurt, or a glass of juice to improve its taste.

**3. Topical Application:

- **Skin Conditions:** For topical application on the skin, a small amount of black seed oil can be applied to affected areas. It's advisable to perform a patch test first to check for any skin sensitivity.

- **Hair and Scalp:** When using black seed oil for hair and scalp health, a small amount can be applied and massaged into the scalp or added to hair care products.

**4. Consultation with Healthcare Professionals:

- **Individual Considerations:** Dosage can vary based on individual factors such as age, weight, overall health, and specific health conditions.

- **Interaction with Medications:** If you are taking medications or have underlying health conditions, it's crucial to consult with healthcare professionals before incorporating black seed oil into your routine, as it may interact with certain medications.

**5. Gradual Introduction:

- **Start Slowly:** If you are new to black seed oil, consider starting with a lower dosage and gradually increasing it as your body adjusts.

- **Monitor Responses:** Pay attention to how your body responds, and if you experience any adverse effects, consult with a healthcare professional.

**6. Adherence to Recommendations:

- **Follow Recommendations:** Follow the recommended dosage guidelines provided by the product or healthcare professional. Avoid exceeding recommended doses unless advised by a healthcare professional.

It's important to emphasize that individual responses to black seed oil can vary, and what works for one person may not work for another. Always seek guidance from healthcare professionals, especially if you are pregnant, nursing, have existing health conditions, or are taking medications. They can provide personalized advice based on your health status and ensure that the use of black seed oil aligns with your overall health goals.

CONCLUSION

In concluding our exploration of black seed oil, we find ourselves at the crossroads of tradition and modern science, a juncture where ancient wisdom meets contemporary inquiry. Throughout this journey, we've delved into the historical tapestry that weaves black seed oil into the fabric of diverse cultures, acknowledging its revered place in traditional medicine and culinary practices.

As we bridge the past and present, it's essential to recognize that black seed oil has not only endured the sands of time but also captured the curiosity of scientific scrutiny. Emerging studies offer glimpses into its potential health benefits, teasing out the intricate dance of bioactive compounds that may hold promise in addressing various health concerns.

From anti-inflammatory and antioxidant properties to potential roles in cardiovascular health, diabetes management, and beyond, black seed oil beckons us to consider its holistic potential. Yet, amidst the intrigue, we tread cautiously, recognizing the need for more robust clinical evidence to fully unravel its therapeutic capacities.

The enigma of black seed oil extends beyond its chemical composition; it resonates with the essence of holistic well-being. Whether applied topically for radiant skin, ingested for internal harmony, or contemplated for its historical significance, black seed oil invites us to engage with health on multiple dimensions.

As we part ways with this exploration, let us carry forward a nuanced perspective—a blend of ancient reverence and modern discernment. Let us celebrate the richness of cultural traditions that have upheld black seed oil, while remaining vigilant in our pursuit of evidence-based understanding. In the realm of health, the journey is ongoing, and the mysteries of nature continue to unfold.

So, here we stand, having traversed the historical landscapes and scientific frontiers of black seed oil. Our conclusions, like the oil itself, are a distillation—a synthesis of tradition and research, an acknowledgment that the story of black seed oil is one that continues to be written. May this exploration inspire curiosity, promote informed choices, and pave the way for a future where ancient remedies and modern insights harmonize in the pursuit of well-being.